THE *Skinny*
30 MINUTE MEALS
RECIPE BOOK

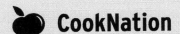
CookNation

THE SKINNY 30 MINUTE MEALS RECIPE BOOK
GREAT FOOD, EASY RECIPES, PREPARED & COOKED IN 30 MINUTES OR LESS. ALL UNDER 300,400 & 500 CALORIES

ISBN 978-1-909855-77-9

A CIP catalogue record of this book is available from the British Library

DISCLAIMER

Some recipes may contain nuts or traces of nuts. Those suffering from any allergies associated with nuts should avoid any recipes containing nuts or nut based oils.

This information is provided and sold with the knowledge that the publisher and author do not offer any legal or other professional advice.

In the case of a need for any such expertise consult with the appropriate professional.

This book does not contain all information available on the subject, and other sources of recipes are available.

This book has not been created to be specific to any individual's requirements.

Every effort has been made to make this book as accurate as possible. However, there may be typographical and or content errors. Therefore, this book should serve only as a general guide and not as the ultimate source of subject information.

This book contains information that might be dated and is intended only to educate and entertain.

The author and publisher shall have no liability or responsibility to any person or entity regarding any loss or damage incurred, or alleged to have incurred, directly or indirectly, by the information contained in this book.

CONTENTS

SKINNY 30 MINUTE SEAFOOD DISHES   65

You may also enjoy.....

DELICIOUS, NUTRITIOUS & SUPER-FAST MEALS IN 15 MINUTES OR LESS. ALL UNDER 300, 400 & 500 CALORIES

ISBN 978-1-909855-42-7

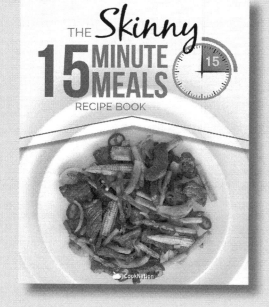

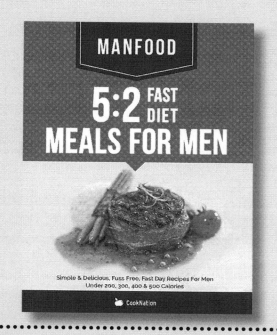

SIMPLE & DELICIOUS, FUSS FREE, FAST DAY RECIPES FOR MEN UNDER 200, 300, 400 & 500 CALORIES

ISBN 978-1-909855-69-4

INTRODUCTION

Perfect for those weekday nights when there just aren't enough hours in the day.

Skinny 30 Minute Meals are perfect for those days when time is not on your side but you still want a delicious, no fuss, low calorie dinner prepared and cooked in under 30 minutes.

Whether you are short of time or perhaps are not experienced in the kitchen and looking for quick and easy recipes, you'll love these simple and speedy suppers. Perfect for those weekday nights when there just aren't enough hours in the day.

What's really great about our skinny 30 minute meals is their simplicity. Each recipe has been carefully created to suit any cook. Many 30 minute recipes use hard to find and often costly ingredients as well as the need for expensive kitchen gadgets. Before you know it every inch of your kitchen space has been taken up before you even start prepping a very tight, pressurised 30 minute recipe.

Our skinny recipes cut out unnecessary ingredients and equipment without compromising on flavour so even the novice chef can create a great tasting weekday supper under 300, 400 or 500 calories.

Our speedy techniques and simple fresh ingredients fast track your meal times. It's the go-to cookbook for busy people who want to create effortless, tasty meals while still keeping track of calories...all in 30 minutes or less.

WHAT DO YOU NEED COOK A MEAL IN UNDER 30 MINUTES?
Cooking meals quickly does require a certain amount of thinking ahead. There are essential store cupboard ingredients that will save you time in the kitchen and of course for speedy prep you will need to use some basic electrical kitchen appliances.

STORE CUPBOARD ESSENTIALS
The following is a list of really handy ingredients to have in your cupboard that you will use over and over again when cooking. Most have a long shelf life and don't need to be kept in the fridge. Building up your store cupboard over time will ensure you always have a dried spice, dash of sauce or stock to hand.

- Tomato puree
- Tomato passata
- Mixed tinned/canned beans
- Lemon juice
- Plain flour
- Cornflour
- Chicken & vegetable stock
- Garlic
- Dried spices : papirka, turmeric, cumin, ginger, coriander, chilli powder, chilli flakes, garam masala
- Curry powder
- Dijon mustard
- Dried Italian herbs: sage, thyme, basil, rosemary, oregano
- Soy Sauce
- Worcestershire sauce
- Tinned chopped tomatoes
- Fresh ginger
- Honey
- Brown sugar
- Salt & pepper

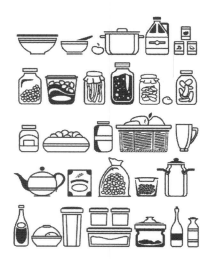

SKINNY FRIDGE ESSENTIALS

To keep calories low, all our recipes apply the skinny factor – that is replacing high calorie/high fat ingredients with lower calorie, healthier alternatives. So if watching your calories is on the agenda when it comes to meal times, then you should always use and have the following in your fridge:

- **Low fat Greek yogurt**
- **Semi skimmed/ half fat milk**
- **Reduced fat cheese**
- **Low fat/unsaturated 'butter' spreads**
- **Low cal cooking oil spray**
- **Low fat cream/ crème fraiche**

SKINNY RECIPES

The recipes in this book are all low calorie dishes for four, which will make it easier for you to monitor your overall daily calorie intake as well as those you are cooking for. The recommended daily calories are approximately 2000 for women and 2500 for men.

Broadly speaking, by consuming the recommended levels of calories each day you should maintain your current weight. Reducing the number of calories (a calorie deficit) will result in losing weight. This happens because the body begins to use fat stores for energy to make up the reduction in calories, which in turn results in weight loss. We have already counted the calories for each dish making it easy for you to fit this into your daily eating plan whether you want to lose weight, maintain your current figure or are just looking for some great-tasting, comforting, winter warming recipes.

I'M ALREADY ON A DIET. CAN I USE THESE RECIPES?

Yes of course. All the recipes can be great accompaniments to many of the popular calorie-counting diets. We all know that sometimes dieting can result in hunger pangs, cravings and boredom from eating the same old foods day in and day out. Skinny 30 Minutes Meals provide filling recipes that should satisfy you for hours afterwards.

I AM ONLY COOKING FOR ONE. WILL THIS BOOK WORK FOR ME?

Yes. We would recommend either following the method for four servings then, where appropriate, dividing and storing the rest for you to use another day. Alternatively divide the quantities by 4 and cook a single meal.

PREPARATION & COOKING TIMES

All the recipes should take no longer than 30 minutes to prepare and cook. All meat should be trimmed of visible fat and the skin removed.

NUTRITION

All of the recipes in this collection are balanced low calorie meals that should keep you feeling full. It is important to balance your food between proteins, good carbs, dairy, fruit and vegetables.

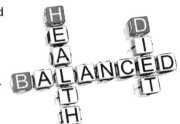

• **Protein**. Keeps you feeling full and is also essential for building body tissue. Good protein sources come from meat, fish and eggs.

• **Carbohydrates**. Not all carbs are good and generally they are high in calories, which makes them difficult to include in a calorie limiting diet. However carbs are a good source of energy for your body as they are converted more easily into glucose (sugar) providing energy. Try to eat 'good carbs' which are high in fibre and nutrients e.g. whole fruits and veg, nuts, seeds, whole grain cereals, beans and legumes.

• **Dairy**. Dairy products provide you with vitamins and minerals. Cheeses can be very high in calories but other products such as low fat Greek yoghurt, crème fraiche and skimmed milk are all good.

• **Fruit & Vegetables.** Eat your five a day. There is never a better time to fill your 5 a day quota. Not only are fruit and veg very healthy, they also fill up your plate and are ideal snacks when you are feeling hungry.

PORTION SIZES

The size of the portion that you put on your plate will significantly affect your weight loss efforts. Filling your plate with over-sized portions will obviously increase your calorie intake and hamper your dieting efforts.

It's important with all meals that you use a correct sized portion, which generally is the size of your clenched fist. This applies to any side dishes of vegetables and carbs too.
The portion sizes in our 30 Minute Meal recipes are the correct size for the average adult but remember that each recipe serves four so don't be tempted to over-fill your plate if you are cooking for one or two!

SKINNY TIPS

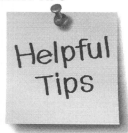

If you are following a diet or generally keeping an eye on your calorie intake, here are some tips that will help you manage the way you eat.

In today's fast moving society many of us have adopted an unhealthy habit of eating. We eat as quickly as possibly without properly giving our bodies the chance to digest and feel full. Not only is this bad for your digestive system, but our bodies begin to relate food to just fuel instead of actually enjoying what we are eating.

Some simple tips for eating which may help you on your fasting days:

- **Eat. Take it slow.** There is no rush.
- **Chew.** It sounds obvious but you should properly chew your food and swallow only when it's broken down and you have enjoyed what you have tasted.
- **Wait.** Before reaching for second helpings wait 5-10 minutes and let your body tell you whether you are still hungry. More often than not, the answer will be no and you will be satisfied with the meal you have had. A glass of water before each meal will help you with any cravings for more.
- **Avoid alcohol** when you can. Alcohol is packed with calories and will counter affect any calorific reduction you are practising with your daily meals.
- **Drink plenty of water** throughout the day. It's good for you, has zero calories, and will fill you up and help stop you feeling hungry.
- **Drink a glass of water before and also with your meal.** Again this will help you feel fuller.
- When you are eating each meal, **put your fork down between bites** – it will make you eat more slowly and you'll feel fuller on less food.
- **Brush your teeth** immediately after your meal to discourage yourself from eating more.
- **If unwanted food cravings do strike, acknowledge them,** then distract yourself. Go out for a walk, phone a friend, play with the kids, or paint your nails.
- **Whenever hunger hits, try waiting 15 minutes** and ride out the cravings. You'll find they pass and you can move on with your day.
- **Remember - feeling a bit hungry is not a bad thing.** We are all so used to acting on the smallest hunger pangs that we forget what it's like to feel genuinely hungry. Learn to 'own' your hunger and take control of how you deal with it.
- **Get moving.** Increased activity will complement your weight loss efforts. Think about what you are doing each day: choose the stairs instead of the lift, walk to the shops instead of driving. Making small changes will not only help you burn calories but will make you feel healthier and more in control of your weight loss.

ALL RECIPES ARE A GUIDE ONLY

All the recipes in this book are a guide only. You may need to alter quantities and cooking times to suit your own appliances.

ABOUT COOKNATION

CookNation is the leading publisher of innovative and practical recipe books for the modern, health conscious cook.

CookNation titles bring together delicious, easy and practical recipes with their unique approach - easy and delicious, no-nonsense recipes - making cooking for diets and healthy eating fast, simple and fun.

With a range of #1 best-selling titles - from the innovative 'Skinny' calorie-counted series, to the 5:2 Diet Recipes collection - CookNation recipe books prove that 'Diet' can still mean 'Delicious'!

Turn to the end of this book to browse all CookNation's recipe books

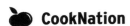 CookNation

Skinny
30 MINUTE MEALS
MEAT DISHES

HONEY KEEMA

405 calories per serving

Ingredients

- 300g/11oz rice
- 1 onion, chopped
- 1 garlic clove, crushed
- 400g/14oz minced/ground turkey
- 200g/7oz frozen peas
- 1 tsp each ground coriander/cilantro & turmeric
- 1 tbsp clear honey
- 2 tbsp soy sauce
- 4 tbsp freshly chopped flat parsley
- Low cal cooking oil spray
- Salt & pepper to taste

Method

1 Cook the rice in a saucepan of salted boiling water for 10-12 minutes or until cooked through. When it's ready, drain and put to one side.

2 Meanwhile in a non-stick frying pan gently sauté the onion & garlic in a little low cal cooking oil for a few minutes until softened. Add the turkey, peas, ground coriander, turmeric, honey & soy sauce to the pan and stir-fry for 5-7 minutes (add a dash of water to the pan if you need to loosen it up).

3 Tip the drained rice into the turkey pan and combine really well continuing to stir-fry until everything is piping hot and cooked through.

4 Sprinkle with chopped parsley and serve.

CHEFS NOTE
Turkey is a great low fat 'skinny' meat option.

SPEEDY CHILLI & RICE

495 calories per serving

Ingredients

- 500g/1lb 2oz lean minced/ground beef
- 1 tsp each ground cumin, coriander/cilantro & paprika
- 400g/14oz tinned chopped tomatoes
- 200g/7oz tinned kidney beans, drained
- 1 tbsp sweet chilli sauce
- 1 tbsp tomato puree/paste
- 200g/7oz rice

- 2 tbsp freshly chopped flat leaf parsley
- Low cal cooking oil spray
- Salt & pepper to taste

Method

1 Heat a little low cal oil in a large high-sided non-stick frying pan and brown the beef for a few minutes.

2 Add all the other ingredients to the pan, except the rice & parsley and combine well.

3 Cover and leave to gently simmer for 15-20 minutes or until everything is cooked through and piping hot.

4 While the chilli is cooking put the rice in a pan of boiling salted water and cook for 10-12 minutes or until the rice is cooked through.

5 Drain the rice and add to the chilli pan, combine well and serve in deep bowls.

CHEFS NOTE
Serve with a handful of plain tortilla chips if you wish.

TERIYAKI CHICKEN

460 calories per serving

Ingredients

- 2 tbsp rice wine
- 4 tbsp soy sauce
- 2 tbsp brown sugar
- 2 tsp freshly grated ginger
- 600g/1lb 5oz chicken breast, cubed
- 2 tsp olive oil
- 250g/9oz rice
- 1lt/4 cups hot vegetable stock

- Low cal cooking oil spray
- Salt & pepper to taste

Method

1 In a bowl mix together the rice wine, soy sauce, brown sugar & ginger. Add the chicken and combine well to coat all the meat.

2 Cook the rice in a saucepan with the stock for 10-12 minutes or until cooked through (add more stock if you need to). When it's ready drain and put to one side.

3 Meanwhile quickly stir-fry the chicken in olive oil for a few minutes until cooked through.

4 Season and serve the chicken piled on top of the rice.

CHEFS NOTE
Serve with freshly chopped chives or spring onions if you like.

SWEET CHICKEN SKEWERS & COUSCOUS

410 calories per serving

Ingredients

- 2 tbsp clear honey
- 2 tbsp soy sauce
- 1 tsp paprika
- 500g/1lb 2oz chicken breast, cubed
- 300g/11oz cherry tomatoes
- 200g/7oz button mushrooms
- 200g/7oz couscous
- 370ml/1½ cups hot chicken stock

- Low cal cooking oil spray
- 8 kebab sticks
- Salt & pepper to taste

Method

1 Preheat the grill.

2 Mix the soy, honey & paprika together and place in a bowl with the chicken, tomatoes & mushrooms. Combine really well to cover everything with the sweet mixture.

3 Place the chicken & vegetables in turn onto the skewers to make kebabs. Place under the grill and cook for 10-12 minutes or until the chicken is cooked through.

4 Meanwhile place the couscous in a bowl with the stock, cover and leave for a few minutes until the stock has absorbed and the couscous is tender.

5 Fluff up with a fork and serve with the cooked skewers.

CHEFS NOTE
Pork or prawns are good with this recipe too.

CORIANDER CHICKEN & PEPPER RICE

450 calories per serving

Ingredients

- 400g/14oz chicken breast, sliced
- 3 tsp ground coriander/cilantro
- 250g/9oz rice
- 1.25lt/5 cups hot vegetable stock
- 1 onion, chopped
- 2 red peppers, deseeded & finely chopped
- 2 garlic cloves, crushed

- 2 medium eggs
- 4 tbsp freshly chopped flat leaf coriander/cilantro
- Low cal cooking oil spray
- Salt & pepper to taste

Method

1 Place the chicken in a plastic bag with the ground coriander and give it a good shake to coat each piece with the spice.

2 Cook the rice in a saucepan with the stock for 10-12 minutes or until cooked through (add more stock if you need to). When it's ready drain and put to one side.

3 Meanwhile gently sauté the onion, peppers & garlic in a little low cal cooking oil for a few minutes until softened. Add the chicken to the pan and stir-fry for 3-4 minutes (add a dash of water to the pan if you need to loosen it up).

4 Tip the drained rice into the chicken pan along with the eggs and stir-fry on a medium heat until the chicken is cooked through and the eggs set into strands.

5 Sprinkle with chopped coriander and serve.

CHEFS NOTE

Add a little spice to the chicken if you like by coating the meat with a pinch of crushed chilli flakes along with the coriander.

CHICKEN & BACON STEW

380 calories per serving

Ingredients

- 500g/1lb 2oz chicken breasts
- 4 slices lean, back bacon, chopped
- 1 onion, chopped
- 2 garlic cloves, crushed
- 400g/14oz tinned chopped tomatoes
- 400g/14oz tinned chickpeas, drained
- 1 tbsp tomato puree/paste
- ½ tsp each salt & brown sugar
- 1 tsp each dried rosemary & paprika
- 120ml/½ cup hot chicken stock
- Low cal cooking oil spray
- Salt & pepper to taste

Method

1 Heat a little low cal oil in a non-stick frying pan and quickly fry the bacon. Add the whole chicken breasts to the pan to seal the meat along with the onions & garlic for a few minutes.

2 Tip this into a saucepan with the chopped tomatoes, chickpeas, puree, salt, sugar, rosemary, paprika & stock. Cover and leave to simmer for 20 minutes.

3 After this time remove the whole chicken breasts and shred them with a couple of forks. Return the meat to the pan and combine well.

4 Season and serve.

CHEFS NOTE
Chicken thighs work well for this recipe too but you will find they are higher in fat than breast meat.

SIMPLE SAUSAGE MEATBALLS

499 calories per serving

Ingredients

- 400g/14oz lean pork sausages
- 1 onion, chopped
- 1 garlic clove, crushed
- 400g/14oz tinned chopped tomatoes
- 500ml/2 cups tomato passata/sauce
- 1 tbsp tomato puree/paste
- ½ tsp each salt & brown sugar
- 200g/7oz fusilli pasta
- Low cal cooking oil spray
- Salt & pepper to taste

Method

1 Slice the top of each sausage open and squeeze the meat out.

2 Use your hands to form the sausage meat into mini meatballs about 2cm/1inch in diameter.

3 Heat a little low cal oil in a non-stick frying pan and gently sauté the onions and garlic for a few minutes until softened. Add the meatballs and move around the pan for a minute or two so that they begin to brown on all sides.

4 Add the tinned tomatoes, passata, puree, salt & sugar to the pan. Combine really well and gently simmer, stirring occasionally, whilst you cook the pasta.

5 Boil the kettle and fill a saucepan with boiling water. Add the pasta and leave to cook for 10-12 minutes or until the fusilli is tender.

6 Check the meatballs are cooked through. Drain the pasta, divide into bowls and load the meatballs & sauce over the top.

CHEFS NOTE

Fusilli is good because it holds the sauce well, but use whichever type of pasta you prefer.

RAGU WITH ORZO

495
calories per
serving

Ingredients

- 1 red onion, finely chopped
- 2 garlic cloves
- 400g/14oz lean mince/ground beef
- 400g/14oz tinned chopped tomatoes
- 250ml/1 cup tomato passata/sauce
- 2 bay leaves
- ½ tsp dried rosemary
- 2 tsp balsamic vinegar

- 300g/11oz orzo pasta
- Low cal cooking oil spray
- Salt & pepper to taste

Method

1 Gently sauté the onion and garlic in a little low cal oil for a few minutes until softened. Add the beef and brown for a further 2-4 minutes.

2 Add the chopped tomatoes, passata, bay leaves, rosemary & balsamic vinegar and simmer for 15 minutes to make a simple ragu.

3 Continue to cook the ragu while you boil the kettle and fill a saucepan with boiling water and a large pinch of salt. Add the pasta and leave to cook for 7-8 minutes or until the orzo is tender.

4 As soon is the pasta is ready quickly drain and add to the ragu.

5 Combine really well, remove the bay leaves, check the seasoning and serve.

CHEFS NOTE

Orzo is a small traditional pasta that cooks more quickly than larger shapes. Feel free to substitute with an alternative if you can't source it.

VIETNAMESE CHICKEN & RICE

455 calories per serving

Ingredients

- 300g/11oz rice
- 1.5lt/6 cups hot vegetable stock
- 4 garlic cloves
- 2 red chillies, deseeded
- ½ tsp crushed sea salt flakes
- 2 tbsp fish sauce
- 1 tbsp caster sugar
- 3 tbsp lime juice
- 400g/14oz cooked chicken breast, shredded
- Large bunch spring onions/scallions, chopped
- Salt & pepper to taste

Method

1 Cook the rice in a saucepan with the stock for 10-12 minutes or until cooked through (add more stock if you need to). When it's ready drain and put to one side.

2 Meanwhile add the garlic, chillies, salt, fish sauce, caster sugar and lime juice to a mini food processor to make the dressing, alter the balance of the dressing to suit your own taste by adding more sugar or lime (if you don't have a food processor just chop everything finely and combine together).

3 When the rice is ready toss the shredded chicken through. Divide into bowls, sprinkle the spring onions over the top and drizzle over the dressing.

CHEFS NOTE

There's plenty of time to grill raw chicken while the rice is cooking if you don't have any pre-cooked chicken to hand.

CHILLI BACON SOUP

200 calories per serving

Ingredients

- 2 onions, chopped
- 2 garlic cloves, crushed
- 125g/5oz bacon, finely chopped
- 1 red chilli deseeded & finely sliced
- 125g/5oz red lentils
- 400g/14oz tinned chopped tomatoes
- 750ml/3 cups hot vegetable stock
- 2 tbsp freshly chopped flat leaf parsley

- Low cal cooking oil spray
- Salt & pepper to taste

Method

1 Use a non-stick saucepan to gently sauté the onion, garlic, bacon & chilli in a little low cal oil for a few minutes until softened.

2 Add the lentils, tomatoes & stock. Stir, cover and cook for 15 minutes or until the lentils are tender.

3 Remove two large ladles of soup and place in a bowl.

4 Put the rest of the soup in a blender and puree to a smooth consistency. Return to the pan along with the reserved unblended soup and continue to cook until everything is piping hot.

5 Check the seasoning and serve with chopped parsley sprinkled over the top.

CHEFS NOTE
Reduce the chilli if you don't want the soup to have too much of a 'kick'.

MISO CHICKEN NOODLE SOUP

270 calories per serving

Ingredients

- 1 onion, chopped
- 1lt/4 cups hot chicken stock
- 2 tbsp miso paste
- 200g/7oz noodles
- 2 pak choi/bok choi shredded
- 1 tbsp soy sauce
- 200g/7oz left-over cooked chicken, shredded
- Low cal cooking oil spray
- Salt & pepper to taste

Method

1 Use a non-stick saucepan to gently sauté the onion in a little low cal oil for a few minutes until softened.

2 Add the stock and miso paste and whisk through to combine the paste into the stock.

3 Add the noodles, pak choi, soy sauce & chicken and cook for 5-6 minutes or until the chicken is piping hot and the noodles are tender.

4 Check the seasoning and serve.

CHEFS NOTE
Feel free to throw any veggies you have to hand into this simple savoury soup.

PASTA WITH SAVOY & BACON

430 calories per serving

Ingredients

- 300g/11oz penne pasta
- 1 tbsp olive oil
- 200g/7oz lean, back bacon, finely chopped
- 1 onion, chopped
- 1 garlic clove, crushed
- 1 savoy cabbage, cored & shredded
- 1 tbsp grated Parmesan cheese
- **Salt & pepper to taste**

Method

1 Boil the kettle and fill a saucepan with boiling water. Add the pasta and leave to cook for 10-12 minutes or until the penne is tender.

2 Heat the olive oil in a high-sided non-stick frying pan and gently sauté the bacon, onions and garlic for a few minutes until the onions soften and the bacon is cooked through (increase the heat a little for a minute or two to brown the bacon if you like).

3 For the last 60 seconds of pasta cooking time add the cabbage to the pasta pan.

4 Drain the pasta & cabbage and add to the bacon pan along with the Parmesan cheese. Toss really well, divide into bowls and serve.

CHEFS NOTE
Use pancetta instead of chopped back bacon if you like.

PORCINI & CHICKEN LINGUINE

435 calories per serving

Ingredients

- 25g/1oz dried porcini mushrooms, chopped
- 2 garlic cloves, crushed
- 1 onion, chopped
- 200g/7oz chicken breasts, sliced
- 120ml/ ½ cup dry white wine
- 2 garlic cloves, crushed
- 2 tbsp low fat crème fraiche

- 300g/11oz spaghetti
- Low cal cooking oil spray
- Salt & pepper to taste

Method

1 Place the porcini mushrooms in a cup with a little warm water and leave to rehydrate for a few minutes.

2 Meanwhile add a little low cal spray to a high-sided non-stick frying pan and gently sauté the onions & garlic for a few minutes until softened.

3 Add the chicken and seal the meat for a minute or two.

4 While this is happening boil the kettle and fill a saucepan with boiling water. Add the pasta and leave to cook for 10-12 minutes or until the spaghetti is tender.

5 As soon as the chicken is sealed add the white wine to the pan and increase the heat. Add the porcini mushrooms and continue to cook for a few minutes until the chicken is cooked through and the wine has reduced by half.

6 Stir the crème fraiche through the chicken. Drain the pasta and add to the pan. Toss really well, divide into bowls and serve.

CHEFS NOTE
Try serving with a little freshly chopped rosemary if you wish.

LEMON CHICKEN NOODLES

410 calories per serving

Ingredients

- 300g/11oz fine egg noodles
- 300g/11oz chicken breast sliced diagonally
- 3 tbsp lemon juice
- Pinch of crushed chilli flakes
- 120ml/½ cup chicken stock
- 1 tsp caster sugar
- 1 tbsp soy sauce
- 1 tsp cornflour
- 6 spring onions/scallions, finely sliced lengthways into ribbons
- Low cal cooking oil spray
- Salt & pepper to taste

Method

1 Place the noodles in boiling water and leave to cook for a few minutes until softened (when they are ready, drain and set to one side).

2 Meanwhile heat a little low cal oil in a wok and stir-fry the chicken strips for a few minutes until cooked through. Turn the heat off for a minute while you make the sauce.

3 Add the lemon juice, chilli flakes, chicken stock, caster sugar and soy sauce to a saucepan and begin warming on a gentle heat. Mix the cornflour in a cup with a little water (1-2 teaspoons a time) to make a paste then add to the saucepan to thicken the sauce.

4 When it's ready add the noodles to the chicken along with the lemon sauce and whack the heat up. Combine everything really well and serve with the spring onion ribbons sprinkled on top.

CHEFS NOTE

The lemon in this recipe is not too overpowering but feel free to add more if that's how you like it.

GREEN BEAN & CHICKEN CURRY

460 calories per serving

Ingredients

- 200g/7oz chicken breast sliced diagonally
- 2 tbsp green Thai curry paste
- 250ml/1 cup low fat coconut milk
- 300g/11oz green beans
- 300g/11oz rice
- Low cal cooking oil spray
- Salt & pepper to taste

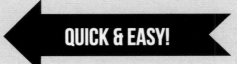

QUICK & EASY!

Method

1 Heat a little low cal oil in a wok and stir-fry the chicken strips for a few minutes.

2 Stir through the Thai curry paste, add the coconut milk along with the green beans and leave to gently simmer.

3 Meanwhile cook the rice in a pan of salted water for 10-12 minutes or until tender.

4 Check the chicken is cooked through. Drain the rice and divide into bowls.

5 Load the curry over the top and serve.

CHEFS NOTE

If you prefer your green beans crunchy hold off adding them to the coconut milk until 2-3 minutes before serving.

CITRUS & HERB RARE SIRLOIN

420 calories per serving

Ingredients

- 800g/1¾lb lean sirloin steak, trimmed
- 2 tbsp extra virgin olive oil
- 2 tsp dried oregano
- 2 garlic cloves, crushed
- Zest of 1 lemon + 2 tsp lemon juice
- ½ tsp salt
- 400g/14oz tenderstem broccoli, sliced in half lengthways
- Salt & pepper to taste

Method

1 Place a high-sided non-stick frying pan on a high heat.

2 Season the steak and brush both sides with a little of the olive oil. Place in the smoking hot pan to cook for 2 minutes each side.

3 Whilst the steak is cooking plunge the broccoli into pan of salted boiling water for 1 minute and drain.

4 Remove the steak from the pan and leave to rest for 2 minutes.

5 Add the rest of the olive oil to the now empty pan and place on a low heat. Add the oregano, garlic, lemon juice, salt & broccoli and gently move around the pan.

6 When the steak has rested use a very sharp knife to thinly slice. Add the slices to the pan. Combine well and serve immediately.

CHEFS NOTE

Sirloin steak is not cheap but it's worth treating yourself now and again! Feel free to 'bulk up' the dish with extra veggies or salad.

CLASSIC PEA & HAM SOUP

295
calories per serving

Ingredients

- 1 onion, chopped
- 300g/11oz potato, peeled & cubed
- 300g/11oz frozen peas
- 750ml/3 cups hot chicken stock
- 250ml/1 cup semi skimmed/half fat milk
- 200g/7oz cooked ham, shredded
- Low cal cooking oil spray
- Salt & pepper to taste

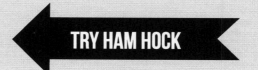

TRY HAM HOCK

Method

1 Use a non-stick saucepan to gently sauté the onion & potato in a little low cal oil for a few minutes until softened.

2 Add the peas & stock and cook for 8-10 minutes or until the potatoes are tender.

3 Use a blender to puree the soup to a smooth consistency. Return to the pan and stir through the milk on a gentle heat. Add the shredded ham and continue to cook until everything is piping hot.

4 Season with lots of black pepper and serve.

CHEFS NOTE
Use thick cut, good quality smoked ham if you can.

CHICKEN & PARSLEY RISOTTO

445 calories per serving

Ingredients

- 2 tbsp olive oil
- 1 onion, chopped
- 2 garlic cloves, crushed
- 300g/11oz risotto rice
- 750ml/3 cups hot chicken stock
- 200g/7oz shredded, cooked chicken
- 4 tbsp freshly chopped flat leaf parsley
- 2 tbsp lemon juice
- 1 egg
- 1 tbsp low fat crème fraiche
- Salt & pepper to taste

Method

1 Heat the olive oil in a high-sided non-stick frying pan and gently sauté the onions & garlic for a few minutes until softened.

2 Add the rice and combine well to coat each grain in the oil. Add a ladleful of stock, stir well and simmer. Repeat until all the stock has been absorbed and/or the rice is tender (add more stock if needed). This should take 15-20 minutes in total, but add the chicken & parsley after 10 minutes.

3 Meanwhile beat together the lemon juice, egg & crème fraiche in a separate bowl. When the risotto is ready stir through the egg mixture and warm for two minutes.

4 Season well and serve.

CHEFS NOTE

If you don't have any pre-cooked chicken to hand, place fresh chicken breasts under the grill and cook for 10 minutes while the risotto is cooking.

BROAD BEAN SPANISH SUPPER

295
calories per serving

Ingredients

- 300g/11oz peas
- 300g/11oz baby broad beans
- 2 tbsp olive oil
- 1 onion
- 2 garlic cloves
- 125g/4oz chorizo, chopped
- 1 tbsp freshly chopped mint
- 2 tsp lemon juice
- Salt & pepper to taste

Method

1 Cook the broad beans & peas in a pan of salted boiling water for 4-6 minutes or until tender. Drain and set to one side.

2 Whilst the beans are cooking heat the olive oil in a non-stick saucepan and gently sauté the onion, garlic & chorizo for a few minutes until softened.

3 Add the drained beans & peas to the pan, stir through the mint & lemon juice and serve with plenty of seasoning.

CHEFS NOTE
Use the youngest, most tender broad beans you can find.

CHINESE PORK MEATBALLS

490 calories per serving

Ingredients

- 300g/11oz rice
- 400g/14oz lean pork mince/ground pork
- 3 slices lean, back bacon, finely chopped
- ½ onion, chopped
- 3 garlic cloves, crushed
- 1 red chilli deseeded & finely shopped
- 1 tbsp lime juice
- 1 tsp ground coriander/cilantro
- ½ tsp ground ginger
- 4 tbsp sweet chilli dipping sauce
- Low cal cooking oil spray
- Salt & pepper to taste

Method

1 Cook the rice in a pan of salted boiling water for 10-12 minutes or until tender. Drain when ready.

2 Meanwhile use a mixer, or your hands, to combine together the meatballs, bacon, onion, garlic, chilli, lime juice, ground coriander & ginger.

3 Use your hands to form the meatball mixture into firm walnut sized balls.

4 Heat a little low cal oil in a non-stick frying pan and stir-fry for 8-12 minutes or until the balls are cooked through and piping hot.

5 Serve the meatballs on top of the drained rice with the chilli sauce drizzled over.

CHEFS NOTE
Make sure the meatball mixture is pressed together firmly as they need to hold together while you are stir-frying them in the pan.

SPICY CHICKEN FAJITAS

399 calories per serving

Ingredients

- 400g/14oz chicken breast, sliced
- 1 tsp each chilli powder, cumin, paprika & garlic powder
- ½ tsp each salt & brown sugar
- 1 red onion, sliced
- 4 red or yellow peppers, deseeded & sliced
- 1 tbsp lime juice

- 4 regular tortilla warps
- 2 baby gem lettuce, shredded
- 4 tbsp fat free Greek yogurt
- Low cal cooking oil spray
- Salt & pepper to taste

Method

1 Place the chicken is a plastic bag with the chilli, cumin, paprika, garlic powder, salt & brown sugar and give it a good shake to coat each piece with the spice.

2 In a non-stick frying pan gently sauté the sliced red onion & peppers in a little low cal cooking oil for a few minutes until softened. Add the chicken to the pan and stir-fry for 3-4 minutes (add a dash of water to the pan if you need to loosen it up).

3 When the chicken is cooked, stir through the lime juice and tip the contents of the frying pan into the flour tortillas along with the shredded lettuce and a dollop of Greek yogurt.

4 Wrap each tortilla up and eat straight away.

CHEFS NOTE
Add some chopped tomatoes and fresh coriander to the fajita wraps too if you like.

JERK CHICKEN & SAVOURY RICE

450 calories per serving

Ingredients

- 400g/14oz chicken breast, thickly sliced
- 2 tsp mixed spice
- 1 tsp each garlic powder & crushed chilli flakes
- 300g/11oz rice
- 1.25lt/5 cups hot vegetable stock
- 200g/7oz peas
- 2 tbsp lime juice
- 4 tbsp freshly chopped flat leaf parsley
- Low cal cooking oil spray
- Salt & pepper to taste

Method

1 Place the chicken is a plastic bag with the mixed spice, garlic powder & crushed chilli flakes and give it a good shake to coat each piece with the spice mixture.

2 Cook the rice in a saucepan with the stock for 10-12 minutes or until cooked through: add more stock if you need to, plus the peas for a few minutes before the end of cooking time.

3 When the rice and peas are both ready drain and put to one side.

4 Meanwhile heat a little low cal cooking oil in a non-stick frying pan and stir-fry the chicken for 3-5 minutes or until the chicken is cooked through (add a dash of water to the pan if you need to loosen it up).

5 Divide the rice into bowls. Stir the lime juice through the chicken and tip over the rice. Sprinkle with chopped parsley and serve.

CHEFS NOTE

This is hot hot hot! Reduce the chilli quantity if you wish.

MUSTARD CHICKEN & LIMA BEAN SALAD

300 calories per serving

Ingredients

- 400g/14oz chicken breast, thickly sliced
- 3 tbsp whole grain mustard
- 2 tbsp olive oil
- 2 tbsp white wine vinegar
- 2 red chilies, deseeded & finely chopped
- 4 tbsp freshly chopped flat leaf parsley
- 300g/11oz tinned lima beans, drained & rinsed
- 1 red onion, very finely sliced
- Salt & pepper to taste

Method

1 Preheat the grill.

2 In a bowl mix together the chicken & mustard and place under the preheated grill. Cook for 6-10 minutes or until cooked through (turning occasionally).

3 Meanwhile toss together the olive oil, vinegar, chillies, parsley, beans and sliced red onion.

4 Divide into bowls and serve the warm mustard chicken over the cold bean salad.

CHEFS NOTE

Substitute tinned black eye beans for lima beans if they are easier to source.

SALT & PEPPER CHICKEN

340 calories per serving

Ingredients

- 1 tbsp olive oil
- 500g/1lb 2oz chicken breast, sliced
- 3 tsp crushed sea salt flakes
- 2 red chillies, deseeded & finely sliced
- ½ tsp brown sugar
- 1 tbsp freshly ground black pepper
- 1 tbsp lime juice
- 1 tsp paprika
- 4 regular sized flat breads
- 4 tbsp fat free Greek yogurt
- Salt & pepper to taste

Method

1 Heat the olive oil in a non-stick frying pan and add the chicken.

2 Stir-fry for 1 minute to seal the meat before adding the salt, chillies, brown sugar, pepper, lime juice & paprika.

3 Cook for 4-5 minutes or until cooked through.

4 Load the chicken into the flat breads along with the yogurt. Season & serve.

CHEFS NOTE

This simple lunch can be bulked up with some salad and/or fresh sliced onions & tomatoes.

Skinny
30 MINUTE MEALS

VEGETABLE DISHES

CUMIN, RUNNER BEAN STEW

SERVES 4

255 calories per serving

Ingredients

- 2 tbsp olive oil
- 1 onion
- 3 garlic cloves, crushed
- 400g/14oz vine ripened tomatoes, chopped
- 4 tsp ground cumin
- 600g/1lb 5oz runner beans, chopped
- 2 tbsp tomato puree/paste
- 1 tsp brown sugar
- 60ml/¼ cup vegetable stock
- Salt & pepper to taste

Method

1 Heat the olive oil in a non-stick saucepan and gently sauté the onion and garlic for a few minutes until softened.

2 Add the tomatoes, cumin, runner beans, puree, sugar and stock. Cover and leave to gently simmer for 15-20 minutes.

3 Season and serve.

CHEFS NOTE
Try serving this veggie dish with rice or crusty bread.

VEGETABLE CHIANG MAI NOODLES

400 calories per serving

Ingredients

- 2 onions, chopped
- 2 garlic cloves, crushed
- 500g/1lb 2oz mixed vegetables
- 500ml/2 cups hot vegetable stock
- 1 tsp turmeric
- ½ tsp each brown sugar & crushed chilli flakes
- 2 tbsp red Thai curry paste
- 200g/7oz fine egg noodles
- 2 tbsp coconut cream
- 1 tbsp lime juice
- 4 tbsp freshly chopped coriander/cilantro
- Low cal cooking oil spray
- Salt & pepper to taste

Method

1 Heat a little low cal oil in a wok and gently sauté the onions & garlic for a few minutes until softened.

2 Add the mixed vegetables to the wok along with the stock, turmeric, sugar, chillies & curry paste and allow to simmer for 5-10 minutes.

3 Meanwhile place the noodles in boiling water. Cover and leave to cook for a few minutes until softened (when they are ready, drain and set to one side).

4 When the vegetables are tender, add the coconut cream, lime juice & noodles and cook in the wok for 5 minutes or until everything is piping hot and cooked through.

5 Sprinkle with chopped coriander and serve.

CHEFS NOTE
Thai curry paste is a really handy store cupboard ingredient to have around.

MINTED PEA & SPINACH RICE

360 calories per serving

Ingredients

- 300g/11oz rice
- 1 tbsp olive oil
- 1 onion
- 2 garlic cloves
- 500g/1lb 2oz petit pois
- 2 tbsp fresh mint, finely chopped
- 150g/5oz spinach leaves
- 250ml/1 cup hot vegetable stock
- Salt & pepper to taste

Method

1 Cook the rice in a saucepan of salted boiling water for 10-12 minutes or until cooked through. When it's ready drain and put to one side.

2 Whilst the rice is cooking heat the olive oil in a wok and gently sauté the onions & garlic for a few minutes until softened.

3 Add the peas, mint and stock to the wok and cook until the peas are tender and the stock disappears. Add the spinach and rice to the pan, toss well and serve.

CHEFS NOTE
This simple veggie dish is great as a side dish for 6 or a meal in it's own right for 4.

GREEN BEANS WITH CAPER DRESSED RICE

440 calories per serving

Ingredients

- 300g/11oz rice
- 1lt/4 cups hot vegetable stock
- 2 tbsp red wine vinegar
- 1 tbsp clear honey
- 3 tbsp olive oil
- 2 tbsp capers, rinsed & chopped
- 15 black pitted olives, sliced

- 400g/14oz green beans, roughly chopped
- Salt & pepper to taste

Method

1 Cook the rice in a saucepan with the stock for 10-12 minutes or until cooked through (add a little more stock to the pan if needed). When it's ready drain and put to one side.

2 Whilst the rice is cooking combine the vinegar, honey, oil & capers to make a dressing.

3 Place the green beans in a pan of salted boing water and cook for 2-3 minutes or until tender. Drain and toss together with the dressing and rice.

4 Season & serve.

CHEFS NOTE
Use pitted green olives if you don't have black olives.

ASPARAGUS & LEMON RISOTTO

385 calories per serving

Ingredients

- 2 tbsp olive oil
- 1 onion, chopped
- 2 garlic cloves, crushed
- 300g/11oz risotto rice
- 750ml/3 cups hot vegetable stock
- 200g/7oz asparagus tips, chopped
- 2 tbsp lemon juice
- Salt & pepper to taste

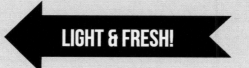

LIGHT & FRESH!

Method

1 Heat the olive oil in a high-sided non-stick frying pan and gently sauté the onions & garlic for a few minutes until softened.

2 Add the rice and combine well to coat each grain in the oil. Add a ladleful of stock, stir well and simmer. Repeat until all the stock has been absorbed and/or the rice is tender (add more stock if needed). This should take 15-20 minutes.

3 When the risotto is almost ready plunge the asparagus into a pan of boiling water for one minute. Drain and add to the risotto.

4 Stir through the lemon juice, season really well and serve.

CHEFS NOTE
Shaved parmesan cheese & rocket leaves make a good addition to this simple risotto.

VEGGIE MISO NOODLES

320 calories per serving

Ingredients

- 1 onion, chopped
- 200g/7oz asparagus tips, roughly chopped
- 150g/5oz mini corn, sliced in half lengthways
- 300g/7oz noodles
- 2 tbsp miso paste
- 4 tbsp boiling water
- 1 tbsp soy sauce
- 1 tbsp lime juice
- Bunch spring onions, scallions, finely chopped
- Low cal cooking oil spray
- Salt & pepper to taste

Method

1 Heat a little low cal oil in a wok and gently sauté the onions, asparagus & mini corn for a few minutes until softened.

2 Meanwhile place the noodles in boiling water and leave to cook for a few minutes until softened (when they are ready, drain and set to one side).

3 Add the miso paste, water & soy sauce to the wok and combine really well so that the miso paste loosens up. Add the warm, cooked noodles & lime juice and continue to stir-fry for a minute or two (add another splash of boiling water if you need to loosen the pan up).

4 Season and serve with the chopped spring onions sprinkled over the top.

CHEFS NOTE
The asparagus and mini corn should still have a little crunch to them. If you prefer them soft, blanch for 1 minute first in boiling water.

DIJON ONION SOUP

120 calories per serving

Ingredients

- 2 tbsp olive oil
- 4 onions, chopped
- ½ tsp brown sugar
- 1 tbsp plain/all purpose flour
- 1 tbsp Dijon mustard
- 1.25lt/5 cups hot chicken stock
- 1 tsp dried mixed herbs
- Salt & pepper to taste

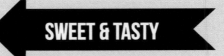

SWEET & TASTY

Method

1 Use a non-stick saucepan to gently sauté the onion & sugar in the olive oil for 15 minutes or until the onions are softened and caramelised.

2 Stir in the flour & mustard and cook for a minute or two before adding the stock and dried herbs.

3 Cook for a further 5-10 minutes, check the seasoning and serve.

CHEFS NOTE
You could use English mustard for this soup, but you'll need to decrease the quantity if you do.

GINGER & SWEET CARROT SOUP

185 calories per serving

Ingredients

- 1 tbsp olive oil
- 2 onions, chopped
- 2 tsp freshly grated ginger
- 800g/1¾lb carrots, chopped
- 2 tsp clear honey
- 1.25lt/5 cups hot vegetable stock
- Salt & pepper to taste

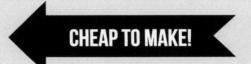

CHEAP TO MAKE!

Method

1 Use a non-stick saucepan to gently sauté the onion & ginger in the olive oil for a few minutes until softened.

2 Add the carrots, honey & stock and cook for 10-12 minutes or until the carrots are tender.

3 Put the soup in a blender and puree to a smooth consistency.

4 Check the seasoning and serve.

CHEFS NOTE
Try serving with a couple of tablespoons of freshly chopped flat leaf parsley or a handful of homemade croutons (see page 64 for recipe).

SPINACH DHAL

Ingredients

- 1 onion, chopped
- 2 garlic cloves, crushed
- 1 tbsp olive oil
- 250g/9oz red lentils
- 1 tsp each ground cumin, coriander/ cilantro, chilli powder, paprika & turmeric
- 1.25lt/5 cups hot vegetable stock
- 300g/11oz spinach leaves

- 4 tbsp fat free Greek yogurt
- Salt & pepper to taste

Method

1 Use a non-stick saucepan to gently sauté the onion & garlic in the olive oil for a few minutes until softened.

2 Add the lentils, spices, stock & spinach. Stir, cover and cook for 15-20 minutes or until the lentils are tender.

3 Place the soup in a blender and puree to a smooth consistency.

4 Divide into bowls and serve with a dollop of Greek yogurt in the middle.

CHEFS NOTE
Alter the consistency of the soup by adding a little more stock if you wish.

CAPER & SHORT SPAGHETTI SOUP

160 calories per serving

Ingredients

- 1 onion, chopped
- 1 celery stalk, sliced
- 1 garlic clove, crushed
- 800g/1¾lb tinned chopped tomatoes
- 75g/3oz pitted black olives, sliced
- 750ml/3 cups hot vegetable stock
- 100g/3½oz spaghetti
- 1 tbsp capers, rinsed & chopped
- Low cal cooking oil spray
- Salt & pepper to taste

Method

1 Use a non-stick saucepan to gently sauté the onion, celery & garlic in a little low cal oil for a few minutes until softened.

2 Add the chopped tomatoes, olives & stock. Break the spaghetti into short lengths and add to the pan.

3 Stir, cover and leave to simmer for 8 minutes or until the spaghetti is cooked through.

4 Stir through the capers and serve.

CHEFS NOTE
Add some crushed dried chillies to this soup if you wish.

HEARTY CHICKPEA & LENTIL SOUP

SERVES 4

240 calories per serving

Ingredients

- 1 onion, chopped
- 125g/5oz red lentils
- 1 tsp each ground cumin & turmeric
- 300g/11oz tinned chickpeas, drained
- 400g/14oz tinned chopped tomatoes
- 750mL/3 cups hot vegetable stock
- Low cal cooking oil spray
- Salt & pepper to taste

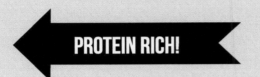

PROTEIN RICH!

Method

1 Use a non-stick saucepan to gently sauté the onion in a little low cal oil for a few minutes until softened.

2 Add the lentils, spices, chickpeas, tomatoes & stock. Stir, cover and cook for 15 minutes or until the lentils are tender.

3 Remove two large ladles of soup and place in a bowl.

4 Put the rest of the soup in a blender and puree the soup to a smooth consistency. Return to the pan along with the reserved unblended soup and continue to cook until everything is piping hot.

5 Season with lots of black pepper and serve.

CHEFS NOTE
Alter the consistency of the soup by adding a little more stock if you wish.

TURMERIC TOMATOES

Ingredients

- 1 tbsp olive oil
- 2 onions, sliced
- 3 garlic cloves, crushed
- 900g/2lb cherry tomatoes, halved
- 2 tsp turmeric
- 1 tsp paprika
- 1 tbsp Dijon mustard
- 300g/11oz frozen peas

- 200g/7oz rice
- Salt & pepper to taste

Method

1 Heat the olive oil in a high-sided non-stick frying pan and gently sauté the onion & garlic in a little low cal cooking oil for a few minutes until softened.

2 Add the tomatoes, turmeric, paprika, mustard & peas and leave to gently simmer for 15 minutes, stirring occasionally.

3 Meanwhile cook the rice in a pan of salted water for 10-12 minutes or until tender.

4 Drain the rice and divide into bowls.

5 Load the tomatoes & peas over the top and serve.

CHEFS NOTE
The tomatoes should be breaking down and beginning to lose their shape after 15 minutes of cooking. Cook for a little longer if you need to.

VEGETABLE & GINGER RAMEN

315 calories per serving

Ingredients

- 1lt/4 cups hot vegetable stock
- 250g/9oz thick udon noodles
- 1 onion, chopped
- 1 tsp brown sugar
- 2 tsp freshly grated ginger
- 1 tbsp soy sauce
- 1 red chilli, deseeded & finely chopped
- 200g/7oz mini sweetcorn, sliced lengthways
- 200g/7oz sugar snap peas
- 200g/7oz mushrooms, sliced
- 2 pak choi/bok choi, shredded
- Salt & pepper to taste

Method

1 Place everything, except the noodles, in a large saucepan. Cover and leave to gently simmer for 6 minutes.

2 Add the noodles and cook for a further 3-4 minutes or until everything is piping hot and cooked through.

3 Divide into bowls and serve.

CHEFS NOTE
Use any mix of vegetables you prefer. Pak choi can be substituted for regular shredded cabbage.

CANNELLINI STIR-FRY

365 calories per serving

Ingredients

- 300g/11oz chicken breast, sliced
- 1 onion, chopped
- 300g/11oz prepared stir-fry vegetables
- 2 garlic cloves, crushed
- 1 tsp freshly grated ginger
- 2 tbsp soy sauce
- 800g/1¾lb tinned cannellini beans, drained & rinsed
- 2 tbsp freshly chopped coriander/ cilantro
- Low cal cooking oil spray
- Salt & pepper to taste

Method

1 Heat a little low cal oil in a wok and stir fry the chicken for a minute or two to seal the meat.

2 Add the onions, vegetables, garlic, ginger & soy sauce and stir-fry for a further 2-3 minutes.

3 Add the beans & coriander and move around the wok for a couple of minutes until everything is piping hot.

4 Divide into shallow bowls and serve.

CHEFS NOTE
Bags of prepared stir-fry vegetables are available everywhere but feel free to shred your own veg if you have the time.

SPEEDY VEGETABLE BIRYANI

320 calories per serving

Ingredients

- 300g/11oz rice
- 1lt/4 cups hot vegetable stock
- 2 tbsp medium curry powder
- 2 carrots, peeled & finely diced
- 200g/7oz peas
- 200g/7oz green beans
- 150g/5oz sweetcorn
- 2 tbsp sultanas
- 1 tbsp chopped coriander/cilantro
- Salt & pepper to taste

Method

1 Cook the rice in a saucepan with the stock and curry powder for 10-12 minutes or until the rice is cooked through (add more stock if you need to). When it's ready drain and return to the pan.

2 Place the vegetables in a large saucepan of water and cook for 5 minutes (or until the carrots are tender), add the sultanas for the last minute of cooking.

3 Drain and add to the pan of rice. Combine well, sprinkle with chopped coriander and serve.

CHEFS NOTE
Use a bag of prepared frozen vegetables if you are short of time.

QUICK & EASY VEGGIE 'KEDGEREE'

450 calories per serving

Ingredients

- 300g/11oz rice
- 1.25lt/5 cups hot vegetable stock
- 2 tbsp medium curry powder
- 8 medium eggs
- 2 tbsp lime juice
- 4 tbsp freshly chopped flat leaf parsley
- Large bunch spring onions, finely sliced
- Salt & pepper to taste

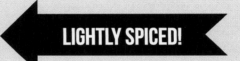

LIGHTLY SPICED!

Method

1 Cook the rice in a saucepan with the stock and curry powder for 10-12 minutes or until the rice is cooked through (add more stock if you need to). When it's ready drain and return to the pan.

2 Meanwhile place the eggs in a saucepan and bring to the boil. Cook for 6 minutes to hard-boil. Drain and place in cold water.

3 Leave the eggs for a minute or two before peeling and cutting into quarters.

4 Add the lime juice to the rice and toss using a fork. Add the egg quarters, parsley & spring onions and gently combine.

5 Season really well and serve.

CHEFS NOTE
Try adding some fresh asparagus tips or spring peas for a little crunch.

ASPARAGUS LAKSA

320 calories per serving

Ingredients

- 250ml/1 cup hot vegetable stock
- 1 onion, chopped
- 1 tsp smooth peanut butter
- 1 tsp freshly grated ginger
- 1 tbsp soy sauce
- 1 tbsp fish sauce
- 2 tsp turmeric
- 2 red peppers, deseeded & finely sliced
- 1 red chilli, deseeded & finely chopped
- 250g/9oz thin rice noodles
- 200g/7oz asparagus tips
- 200g/7oz green beans
- 1 tbsp coconut cream
- Salt & pepper to taste

Method

1 Place everything, except the noodles, asparagus, green beans & coconut cream, in a large saucepan. Cover and leave to gently simmer for 4 minutes.

2 Meanwhile place the noodles in a bowl of boiling water, cover and leave to gently soften. When they are ready drain and add to the saucepan along with the green beans, asparagus & coconut cream.

3 Cook for 2 minutes until the green beans and asparagus are tender. Divide into bowls and serve.

CHEFS NOTE
Try serving with some fresh lime wedges.

CHICKPEAS & HALLOUMI

360 calories per serving

Ingredients

- 1 tbsp olive oil
- 2 red chillies, deseeded & finely chopped
- 1 onion, chopped
- 2 garlic cloves, crushed
- 400g/14oz cherry tomatoes, halved
- 800g/1¾lb tinned chickpeas, drained & rinsed
- 60ml/¼ cup hot vegetable stock
- 125g/4oz halloumi cheese, chopped
- 1 tbsp lemon juice
- 100g/3½oz rocket
- Salt & pepper to taste

Method

1 Heat the olive oil in a high-sided non-stick frying pan and gently sauté the chillies, onion & garlic for a few minutes until softened.

2 Add the cherry tomatoes and cook for 3-4 minutes longer before adding the chickpeas, stock and halloumi. Cover and leave to simmer for 5 minutes.

3 Stir through the lemon juice, toss in the rocket, divide into bowls and serve.

CHEFS NOTE
As Halloumi is free from rennet it is usually suitable for most vegetarians.

FRESH TOMATO LINGUINE

375
calories per serving

Ingredients

- 800g/1¾lb vine ripened tomatoes
- 3 garlic cloves, crushed
- 3 tbsp freshly chopped basil
- ½ tsp each salt & brown sugar
- 2 tbsp olive oil
- 300g/11oz linguine
- Salt & pepper to taste

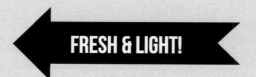

FRESH & LIGHT!

Method

1 Boil the kettle and fill a saucepan with boiling water and a large pinch of salt. Add the pasta and leave to cook for 10-12 minutes or until the linguine is tender.

2 Meanwhile plunge the tomatoes into a bowl of boiling water for 1 minute. Drain and quickly refresh in cold water. Remove each in turn and peel the skins.

3 Roughly chop the peeled tomatoes and combine with the garlic, basil, salt, sugar & olive oil.

4 Your pasta should be ready by now so quickly drain and return to the saucepan. Add the fresh chopped tomatoes and toss really well.

5 Divide into bowls and serve.

CHEFS NOTE

You might find the tomatoes easier to peel if you make a knick in the top of each one with a knife before plunging into the boiling water.

MUSHROOM & THYME PASTA

370 calories per serving

Ingredients

- 1 tbsp olive oil
- 300g/11oz mushrooms, sliced
- 1 onion, chopped
- 2 garlic cloves, crushed
- 1 tsp dried thyme
- 1 tbsp lemon juice
- 300g/11oz spaghetti
- 1 tbsp grated Parmesan cheese
- Salt & pepper to taste

Method

1 Boil the kettle and fill a saucepan with boiling water and a large pinch of salt. Add the pasta and leave to cook for 10-12 minutes or until the spaghetti is tender.

2 Meanwhile heat the olive oil in a high-sided non-stick frying pan and gently sauté the mushrooms, onions, garlic & thyme for 8-10 minutes or until the mushrooms are cooked through.

3 Your pasta should be ready by now so quickly drain and add to the mushroom pan along with the lemon juice.

4 Toss really well, divide into bowls and serve with the grated Parmesan sprinkled over the top.

CHEFS NOTE
Use whichever closed cup mushrooms you have to hand for this recipe.

ITALIAN MIXED BEAN STEW

390 calories per serving

Ingredients

- 1 onion, chopped
- 2 garlic cloves, crushed
- 200g/7oz mushrooms, sliced
- 200g/7oz cherry tomatoes, chopped
- 400g/14oz tinned borlotti beans, drained
- 400g/14oz tinned flageolet beans, drained
- 250ml/1 cup tomato passata/sauce
- 1 tbsp tomato puree/paste
- 2 tbsp freshly chopped flat leaf parsley
- Low cal cooking oil spray
- Salt & pepper to taste

Method

1 Heat a little low cal oil in a high-sided non-stick frying pan and gently sauté the onions, garlic, mushrooms & cherry tomatoes for a few minutes until softened.

2 Add the tinned beans, passata & puree to the pan. Combine really well, cover and leave to gently simmer for about 15 minutes or until everything is piping hot.

3 Season with plenty of salt and pepper, sprinkle with parsley & serve.

CHEFS NOTE
Use any type of tinned bean you prefer for this recipe.

SWEET POTATO & MANGO CURRY

499 calories per serving

Ingredients

- 1 onion, chopped
- 2 tbsp red Thai curry paste
- 120ml/½ cup low fat coconut milk
- 250ml/1 cup hot vegetable stock
- 2 tsp fish sauce
- 300g/11oz sweet potato, peeled & cubed
- 400g/14oz butternut squash, peeled & cubed

- 200g/7oz rice
- 1 tsp lime juice
- 100g/3½oz spinach roughly chopped
- 1 small ripe mango, peeled, de-stoned & cubed
- Low cal cooking oil spray
- Salt & pepper to taste

Method

1 Heat a little low cal oil in a wok and gently sauté the onions for a few minutes until softened. Stir through the Thai curry paste, add the coconut milk, stock & fish sauce.

2 Add the cubed sweet potato & squash and leave to gently simmer for 10-15 minutes or until the tender.

3 While the potatoes are cooking place the rice in a pan of salted boiling water and cook for 10-12 minutes or until tender.

4 Add the lime juice, spinach and mango to the curry and warm through for 2 minutes. Drain the rice and divide into bowls.

5 When the curry is piping hot load over the top of the rice and serve.

CHEFS NOTE

If you are using an under-ripe mango you'll need to cook it for a little longer.

HARICOT & PASTA SOUP

300
calories per serving

Ingredients

- 1 onion, chopped
- 2 celery stalks, chopped
- 2 garlic cloves, crushed
- 300g/11oz carrots, peeled & chopped
- 300g/11oz sweet potato, peeled & cubed
- 1 tsp dried mixed herbs
- 75g/3oz macaroni pasta
- 1lt/4 cups hot vegetable stock

- 400g/14oz tinned haricot beans
- Low cal cooking oil spray
- Salt & pepper to taste

Method

1 Use a non-stick saucepan to gently sauté the onion, celery & garlic in a little low cal oil for a few minutes until softened.

2 Add the carrots, sweet potatoes & herbs and cook for 5 minutes longer (add a splash of water to the pan if you need to loosen it up).

3 Add the pasta & stock and cook for 8 minutes. Add the beans and cook for a further 4-6 minutes or until the pasta and vegetables are tender and piping hot.

CHEFS NOTE
Use any mix of vegetables you have to hand for this hearty veggie soup.

BBQ BEAN & SPINACH ONE-POT

380 calories per serving

Ingredients

- 1 onion, chopped
- 2 garlic cloves, crushed
- 400g/14oz tinned butter beans, drained
- 400g/14oz tinned flageolet beans, drained
- 400g/14oz tinned chopped tomatoes
- 5 tbsp BBQ sauce
- 200g/7oz spinach
- Low cal cooking oil spray
- Salt & pepper to taste

Method

1 Heat a little low cal oil in a high-sided non-stick frying pan and gently sauté the onions & garlic for a few minutes until softened.

2 Add the tinned beans, tomatoes & BBQ sauce to the pan. Combine really well, cover and leave to gently simmer for about 15 minutes or until everything is piping hot and you are left with a thick stew.

3 Add the spinach and cook just long enough to wilt the leaves.

4 Season and serve.

CHEFS NOTE
Use any type of regular shop bought BBQ sauce, the Jack Daniels brand is particularly good.

HOMEMADE CROUTONS

50 calories per portion

Ingredients

- 4 slices thick whole meal bread
- 2 tsp garlic powder
- 2 tsp dried mixed herbs
- 1 tsp crushed sea salt flakes
- Low cal cooking oil spray

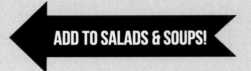

ADD TO SALADS & SOUPS!

Method

1 Preheat the oven to 350f/180c/Gas 4

2 Remove the crusts with a knife and cube the bread into crouton sized pieces.

3 Spray the bread cubes with some low cal spray and place in a plastic bag with the garlic powder, herbs and salt. Give the bag a good shake until all the bread is covered with the seasoning.

4 Lay the bread cubes out on a non-stick baking tray and cook in the preheated oven for 13-15 minutes or until the croutons are crisp and golden brown.

5 Allow to cool. Use straightway or store in an airtight container for up to 3 days.

CHEFS NOTE

You could add some grated Parmesan to the seasoning bag for extra taste.

Skinny
30 MINUTE MEALS

SEAFOOD DISHES

'FANCY' EGG FRIED RICE

440
calories per serving

Ingredients

- 300g/11oz rice
- 1.5lt/6 cups hot vegetable stock
- 1 tbsp olive oil
- 2 onions, sliced
- 4 garlic cloves
- 1 red chilli, deseeded & finely chopped
- 2 tbsp soy sauce

- 400g/14oz raw king prawns/jumbo shrimp, chopped
- 2 medium eggs
- Bunch spring onions/scallions, chopped
- Salt & pepper to taste

Method

1 Cook the rice in a saucepan with the stock for 10-12 minutes, or until cooked through (add more stock if you need to). When it's ready, drain and put to one side.

2 Meanwhile heat the olive oil in a wok and gently sauté the onions, garlic & chilli for a few minutes until softened.

3 Add the soy sauce & prawns and stir-fry before adding the drained rice. Beat the eggs in a cup and add this to the pan too. Stir-fry until the eggs set into strands.

4 Divide into bowls, sprinkle with spring onions and serve.

CHEFS NOTE
Pork, chicken and mixed vegetables are good stir-fried through this rice too.

SIMPLE SWEET CHILLI SALMON

430 calories per serving

Ingredients

- 300g/11oz rice
- 4 skinless salmon fillets, each weighing 150g/5oz
- 2 tbsp sweet chilli sauce
- 1lt/4 cups boiling chicken stock
- Low cal cooking oil spray
- Salt & pepper to taste

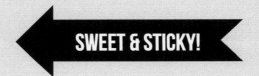

SWEET & STICKY!

Method

1 Smother the salmon fillets in chilli sauce.

2 Cook the rice in a saucepan with the stock for 10–12 minutes or until tender (add more stock if you need to).

3 Meanwhile add a little low cal oil to a non-stick frying pan and place on a high heat. Add the salmon fillets to the smoking hot pan and cook for 2-3 minutes each side (or until cooked though).

4 Drain the rice and divide into bowls. Use a fork to break up the salmon and arrange the flakes over the top of the rice.

CHEFS NOTE
Keep extra sweet chilli sauce on hand to add to the meal when eating.

SCALLOPS & CHICKPEAS

370
calories per serving

Ingredients

- 800g/1¾lb tinned chickpeas
- 2 tbsp freshly chopped flat leaf parsley
- ½ tsp salt
- 100g/3½oz rocket
- 4 tsp olive oil
- 500g/1lb 2oz prepared scallops
- 1 tbsp lemon juice
- Lemon wedges to serve
- Salt & pepper to taste

Method

1 Drain and rinse the chickpeas and combine these with the parsley, salt, rocket & half of the olive oil.

2 Heat the remaining olive oil in a non-stick frying pan. Add the prepared scallops and cook for 1-2 minutes each side (or until cooked through).

3 Add the lemon juice and cook for 30 seconds longer, moving the scallops around the bubbling lemon juice.

4 Tip the scallops out onto a plate and serve with the chickpea salad and lemon wedges

CHEFS NOTE
Try adding some finely sliced chillies to the scallops when cooking.

SPICED SEAFOOD CHOWDER

330 calories per serving

Ingredients

- 1 onion, chopped
- 1 red chilli, deseeded & finely chopped
- 400g/14oz potatoes, peeled & cubed
- 200g/7oz sweetcorn
- 200g/7oz sugar snap peas, roughly chopped
- 1lt/4 cups hot chicken or fish stock
- 300g/11oz raw shelled prawns/shrimp, chopped
- 250ml/1 cup low fat coconut milk
- 1 tbsp lime juice
- Salt & pepper to taste

Method

1 Gently simmer the onions, chilli, potatoes, sweetcorn & peas in the hot chicken stock for 8-10 minutes or until the potatoes are tender.

2 Add the prawns & coconut milk and continue to cook for 3-5 minutes or until the prawns are cooked through.

3 Stir through the lime juice, check the seasoning and serve.

CHEFS NOTE
You could also make this simple chowder using shredded chicken.

SWEET CHILLI PRAWNS & NOODLES

320 calories per serving

Ingredients

- 200g/7oz fine egg noodles
- 1 onion, chopped
- 2 garlic cloves, crushed
- 1 tsp freshly grated ginger
- 200g/7oz peas
- 400g/14oz raw, peeled king prawns/ jumbo shrimp
- 1 tbsp soy sauce
- 2 tbsp sweet chilli sauce
- 1 bunch spring onions/scallions finely chopped
- Low cal cooking oil spray
- Salt & pepper to taste

Method

1 Place the noodles in boiling water and leave to cook for a few minutes until softened (when they are ready, drain and set to one side).

2 Meanwhile heat a little low cal oil in a wok and gently sauté the onions, garlic, ginger & peas for a few minutes until softened (if you are using frozen peas boil for a couple of minutes first).

3 Increase the heat, add the prawns & soy sauce and cook for 5-8 minutes or until the prawns are pink and cooked through. Stir through the sweet chilli sauce and add the noodles to the pan.

4 Stir-fry for a minute or two, sprinkle with the chopped spring onions and serve.

CHEFS NOTE
Serve with prawn crackers if you like, but watch the extra calories!

SIMPLE FISH STEW WITH COUSCOUS

355 calories per serving

Ingredients

- 1 onion, chopped
- 2 garlic cloves, crushed
- 600g/1lb 5oz boneless, white fish fillets
- 500ml/2 cups tomato passata/sauce
- Pinch of dried crushed chillies
- ½ tsp each salt & brown sugar
- 200g/7oz couscous
- 370ml/1½ cups hot chicken stock

- Low cal cooking oil spray
- Salt & pepper to taste

Method

1 Heat a little low cal oil in a non-stick frying pan and gently sauté the onion and garlic for a few minutes until softened.

2 Add the fish, passata, chillies, salt & sugar and cook for 10-15 minutes (add a little chicken stock to the pan if the passata doesn't cover the fillets). Stir occasionally to encourage the fillets to break up a little.

3 Meanwhile place the boiling stock and couscous in a bowl. Cover and leave for 3-4 minutes or until the stock is absorbed. Fluff with a fork and divide into shallow bowls. Serve with the fish stew ladled over the top.

CHEFS NOTE
You may need a little more salt/sugar to balance the acidity of the tomato passata.

SPICED SALMON FILLETS

395 calories per serving

Ingredients

- 4 skinless salmon fillets, each weighing 150g/5oz
- 1 tbsp medium curry powder
- ½ tsp each salt & brown sugar
- 200g/7oz fine egg noodles
- 750ml/3 cups boiling chicken stock
- 1 tbsp soy sauce
- 1 tbsp lime juice
- 1 tbsp fish sauce
- 2 tbsp freshly chopped coriander/cilantro
- Low cal cooking oil spray
- Salt & pepper to taste

Method

1 Mix the curry powder, salt & sugar together in a plastic bag along with the salmon fillets and give everything a good shake to evenly cover the fish in the spices.

2 Place the noodles in the boiling stock and leave to cook for a few minutes (when they are ready, drain and set to one side).

3 Meanwhile add a little low cal oil to a non-stick frying pan and place on a high heat. Add the salmon fillets to the smoking hot pan and cook for 2-3 minutes each side (or until cooked though).

4 In a separate pan, or wok, combine the cooked noodles with the soy sauce, lime juice & fish sauce and gently warm through.

5 Tip the noodles onto plates and place the cooked salmon on top. Sprinkle with coriander and serve.

CHEFS NOTE
Add some cooked shredded cabbage and mini sweetcorn to the noodles too if you like.

FRESH TUNA & SWEET BEAN SALAD

450 calories per serving

Ingredients

- 4 skinless salmon fillets, each weighing 150g/5oz
- 2 tsp lime juice
- 1 tbsp extra virgin olive oil
- ½ red chilli, deseeded & finely chopped
- 1 tsp clear honey
- 2 tbsp freshly chopped flat leaf parsley
- ½ tsp salt

- 800g/1¾lb tinned flageolet beans
- 1 red onion, finely sliced
- 200g/7oz cherry tomatoes, quartered
- Salt & pepper to taste

Method

1 Mix together the lime juice, olive oil, chopped chilli, honey, parsley & salt to make a dressing.

2 Drain & rinse the flageolet beans and toss these with the dressing along with the red onion & cherry tomatoes. Season with plenty of black pepper

3 Place a non-stick frying pan on a high heat. Add the tuna to the smoking hot pan and cook for 1 minute each side (or more if the steaks are thick).

4 Serve the tuna steaks with the bean salad on the side.

CHEFS NOTE

Fresh tuna is best served rare but feel free to alter the cooking time to suit your own taste.

FRESH TUNA PASTA

Ingredients

- 500g/1lb 2oz fresh tuna steaks
- 3 tbsp olive oil
- 1 onion, chopped
- ½ red chilli, deseeded & finely chopped
- 3 garlic cloves, crushed
- 2 tbsp lemon juice
- 2 tbsp freshly chopped basil
- 250g/9oz penne pasta

- 1 lemon, cut into wedges
- Salt & pepper to taste

Method

1 Fill a saucepan with boiling water and a large pinch of salt. Add the pasta and leave to cook for 10-12 minutes or until the penne is tender.

2 Meanwhile heat 1 tbsp of the olive oil in a non-stick frying pan and gently sauté the onions, garlic & chilli for a few minutes until softened.

3 Tip these out onto a plate, increase the heat and cook the tuna steaks in the same pan for 1-2 minutes each side (1 minute if you like it rare). Remove from the pan and place on a chopping board. Use two forks to pull the steaks apart – they meat should naturally flake and come apart in slices.

4 Under a gentle heat add the onions back to the pan along with the rest of the olive oil, lemon juice, chopped basil & tuna slices.

5 Your pasta should be ready by now so quickly drain and add to the tuna pan. Combine really well and serve immediately with lemon wedges.

CHEFS NOTE

Try a different twist on this meal by adding two tablespoons of balsamic vinegar to the pan when you cook the tuna.

PANGRITATA SPAGHETTI

465 calories per serving

Ingredients

- 2 slices brown bread
- 2 garlic cloves
- 1 tsp dried thyme
- 3 tbsp olive oil
- 1 onion, chopped
- 8 tinned anchovy fillets, drained
- 300g/11oz spaghetti

- 1 lemon, cut into wedges
- Salt & pepper to taste

Method

1 Place the bread, garlic & thyme in a food processor along with a good pinch of salt and pulse for a few seconds until the bread turns into breadcrumbs.

2 Gently warm the olive oil in a high-sided non-stick frying pan (reserve 1 tsp of the olive oil for later) and add the breadcrumbs. Move them around the pan to coat well in olive oil and cook for about 5 minutes or until the breadcrumbs gently brown and become crispy turning into pangritata.

3 Meanwhile fill a saucepan with boiling water and a large pinch of salt. Add the pasta and leave to cook for 10-12 minutes or until the spaghetti is tender.

4 When the breadcrumbs are ready tip them out onto a plate to cool.

5 Wipe out the pan with kitchen roll. Add the reserved tsp of olive oil and gently sauté the onions and anchovy fillets for a few minutes until the onions soften and the anchovy fillets break up.

6 Your pasta should be ready by now so quickly drain and add to the anchovy pan. Combine really well and divide into bowls, sprinkle the pangritata over the spaghetti and serve immediately with lemon wedges.

FRESH HERB & SHRIMP FETTUCCINE

415 calories per serving

Ingredients

- 1 tbsp olive oil
- 1 onion, chopped
- ½ red chilli, deseeded & finely chopped
- 2 garlic cloves, crushed
- 2 tbsp lemon juice
- 500g/1lb 2oz raw, peeled king prawns/ jumbo shrimp
- 2 tbsp each freshly chopped flat leaf

- parsley & basil
- 300g/11oz fettuccine
- 1 lemon, cut into wedges
- Salt & pepper to taste

Method

1 Fill a saucepan with boiling water and a large pinch of salt. Add the pasta and leave to cook for 10-12 minutes or until the fettuccine is tender.

2 Meanwhile heat the olive oil in a high-sided non-stick frying pan and gently sauté the onions, garlic & chilli for a few minutes until softened.

3 Add the lemon juice and prawns and cook for about 5-7 minutes or until the prawns are pink and cooked through.

4 Your pasta should be ready by now so quickly drain and add to the prawn pan.

5 Combine everything together, sprinkle in the chopped fresh herbs and toss really well.

6 Divide into bowls and serve immediately with lemon wedges.

CHEFS NOTE
Use whichever mix of fresh herbs you prefer. Chives and rosemary work well together too.

SARDINE & OLIVE PASTA

470 calories per serving

Ingredients

- 300g/11oz spaghetti
- 1 tbsp olive oil
- 250g/9oz tinned sardines (in tomato sauce)
- 1 red onion, sliced
- 2 garlic cloves, crushed
- 1 tbsp capers, chopped
- 10 black pitted olives, sliced
- Salt & pepper to taste

Method

1 Fill a saucepan with boiling water and a good pinch of salt. Add the pasta and leave to cook for 10-12 minutes or until the spaghetti is tender.

2 Meanwhile heat the olive oil in a high-sided non-stick frying pan and gently sauté the sardines, onions, garlic, capers & olives for 10-15 minutes or until everything is cooked through and piping hot.

3 Drain the pasta and add to the sardine pan. Toss really well, divide into bowls and serve.

CHEFS NOTE
This is a super easy store cupboard meal you can rustle up in minutes.

PRAWN THAI NOODLES

400 calories per serving

Ingredients

- 300g/11oz fine egg noodles
- 1 onion, chopped
- 2 garlic cloves, crushed
- 1 tsp freshly grated ginger
- 1 red chilli, deseeded & finely chopped
- 400g/14oz raw, peeled king prawns/ jumbo shrimp
- 1 tbsp soy sauce

- 1 tbsp lime juice
- 1 tbsp fish sauce
- 1 medium egg, lightly beaten with a fork
- 2 tbsp freshly chopped coriander/ cilantro
- Low cal cooking oil spray
- Salt & pepper to taste

Method

1 Place the noodles in boiling water and leave to cook for a few minutes until softened (when they are ready, drain and set to one side).

2 Meanwhile heat a little low cal oil in a wok and gently sauté the onions, garlic, ginger & chilli for a few minutes until softened.

3 Increase the heat, add the prawns and cook for 4-7 minutes or until the prawns are pink and cooked through.

4 Add the soy sauce, lime juice & fish sauce and continue to stir fry. Add the noodles along with the egg and stir fry for a few minutes until the egg strands are set and everything is piping hot.

5 Sprinkle with chopped coriander and serve.

CHEFS NOTE
Alter the balance of lime and fish sauce to suit your on taste.

SMOKED FISH & BORLOTTI BEANS

385 calories per serving

Ingredients

- 500g/1lb 2oz smoked boneless haddock or cod fillets
- 500ml/2 cups hot chicken or fish stock
- 800g/1¾lb tinned borlotti beans, drained & rinsed
- 1 tbsp extra virgin olive oil
- 2 tbsp freshly chopped flat leaf parsley
- Salt & pepper to taste

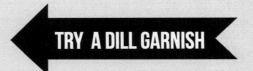

TRY A DILL GARNISH

Method

1 Heat the stock in a high-sided non-stick frying pan and gently poach the fish fillets for 4-5 minutes or until cooked through.

2 Leaving the poaching liquid in the pan remove the fish fillets, wrap them in foil to keep them warm and put to one side.

3 Add the drained borlotti beans to the poaching liquid and cook for 4-5 minutes until piping hot.

4 Drain the beans and return them to the empty pan. Flake the fish and add to the beans along with the oil and parsley.

5 Combine gently, season with lots of black pepper and serve.

CHEFS NOTE
Keep a little extra stock on hand in case you need more to cover the fillets or beans when poaching.

SCALLOPS & SMASHED PEAS

290 calories per serving

Ingredients

- 600g/1lb 5oz frozen peas
- 1 tbsp Thai green curry paste
- 1 tbsp low fat crème fraiche
- ½ tsp salt
- 1 tbsp low fat 'butter' spread
- 500g/1lb 2oz prepared scallops
- 2 tbsp lime juice
- 150g/5oz rocket
- Salt & pepper to taste

Method

1 Cook the frozen peas in a pan of boiling water for a few minutes until tender. When they are ready drain, return to the pan and add the curry paste, crème fraiche & salt. Using a potato masher, or the back of a fork smash up the peas. Cover the pan and put to one side.

2 Heat the 'butter' in a non-stick frying pan. Add the prepared scallops and cook for 1-2 minutes each side (or until cooked through).

3 Add the lime juice and cook for 30 seconds longer, moving the scallops around the bubbling lime juice.

4 Tip the scallops out onto a plate and serve with the smashed peas & rocket on the side.

CHEFS NOTE
Use an olive based low fat 'butter' spread.

PINEAPPLE & PRAWN KEBABS

340 calories per serving

Ingredients

- 500g/1lb 2oz large, shelled king prawns
- 2 tsp lime juice
- 250g/9oz fresh pineapple, cubed
- 3 tbsp desiccated coconut
- 200g/7oz couscous
- 370ml/1½ cups hot chicken stock
- Low cal cooking oil spray
- 8 kebab sticks
- Salt & pepper to taste

Method

1 Preheat the grill.

2 Quickly mix the prawns with the lime juice.

3 Place the prawns & pineapple chunks in turn onto the skewers to make kebabs.

4 Sprinkle the desiccated coconut all over the kebabs. Place under the grill and cook for 8-10 minutes or until the prawns are cooked through.

5 Meanwhile place the couscous in a bowl with the stock, cover and leave for a few minutes until the stock has absorbed and the couscous is tender.

6 Fluff up with a fork and serve with the cooked skewers.

CHEFS NOTE

Use tinned pineapple chunks if you don't have fresh pineapple.

Skinny 30 MINUTE MEALS STOCK RECIPES

Using homemade stock makes a good addition to any meal but it's not a 30 minute job! You'll need to prepare the stock in advance and freeze it in 250ml/1 cup batches.

If you decide to use shop bought stock (which most people do) avoid buying budget options and anything too high in sodium.

If you want to have a go at making stock from scratch here are a few simple recipes to start with. Use the largest saucepan you can find.

BASIC VEGETABLE STOCK

Ingredients

- 1 tbsp olive oil
- 1 onion, chopped
- 1 leek, chopped
- 1 carrot, chopped
- 1 small bulb fennel, chopped
- 3 garlic cloves, crushed
- 1 tbsp black peppercorns
- 75g/3oz mushrooms

- 2 sticks celery, chopped
- 3 tomatoes, diced
- 2 tbsp freshly chopped flat leaf parsley
- 2 bay leaves
- 3lt/12 cups water

Method

Gently sauté the onions, leeks, carrots and fennel in the olive oil for a few minutes in a large lidded saucepan. Add all the other ingredients, cover and bring to the boil. Leave to gently simmer for 30 minutes with the lid on. Allow to cool for a little while. Pour the contents through a sieve and store the finished stock liquid in the fridge for a couple of days or freeze in batches.

BASIC CHICKEN STOCK

Ingredients

- 1 tbsp olive oil
- 1 left over roast chicken carcass
- 2 carrots, chopped
- 2 onions, halved
- 2 stalks celery, chopped
- 10 black peppercorns
- 2 bay leaves
- 2 tbsp freshly chopped parsley

- 1 tsp freshly chopped thyme
- 3lt/12 cups water

Method

Gently sauté the onions, carrots and celery in the olive oil for a few minutes in a large lidded saucepan. Break the chicken carcass up into pieces and add to the pan along with all the other ingredients, cover and bring to the boil. Leave to simmer very gently for 1hr with the lid on. Allow to cool for a little while. Pour the contents through a sieve and store the finished stock liquid in the fridge for a couple of days or freeze in batches. You may find you need to skim a little fat from the top of the stock after cooking.

BASIC FISH STOCK

Ingredients

- 1 tbsp olive oil
- 450g/1lb fish bones, heads carcasses etc. (avoid oily fish when making stock)
- 4 leeks, chopped
- 1 fennel bulb, chopped
- 4 carrots, chopped
- 2 tbsp freshly chopped parsley
- 250ml/1 cup dry white wine

- 2.5lt/10 cups water

Method

Gently sauté the carrots, leeks and fennel in the olive oil for a few minutes in a large lidded saucepan. Clean the fish bones to ensure there is no blood as this can 'spoil' the stock. Add all the other ingredients, cover and bring to the boil. Leave to simmer very gently for 1hr with the lid on. Allow to cool for a little while. Pour the contents through a sieve and store the finished stock liquid in the fridge for a couple of days or freeze in batches. You may find you need to skim a little fat from the top of the stock after cooking.

CONVERSION CHART: DRY INGREDIENTS

Metric	Imperial
7g	¼ oz
15g	½ oz
20g	¾ oz
25g	1 oz
40g	1½oz
50g	2oz
60g	2½oz
75g	3oz
100g	3½oz
125g	4oz
140g	4½oz
150g	5oz
165g	5½oz
175g	6oz
200g	7oz
225g	8oz
250g	9oz
275g	10oz
300g	11oz
350g	12oz
375g	13oz
400g	14oz

Metric	Imperial
425g	15oz
450g	1lb
500g	1lb 2oz
550g	1¼lb
600g	1lb 5oz
650g	1lb 7oz
675g	1½lb
700g	1lb 9oz
750g	1lb 11oz
800g	1¾lb
900g	2lb
1kg	2¼lb
1.1kg	2½lb
1.25kg	2¾lb
1.35kg	3lb
1.5kg	3lb 6oz
1.8kg	4lb
2kg	4½lb
2.25kg	5lb
2.5kg	5½lb
2.75kg	6lb

CONVERSION CHART: LIQUID MEASURES

Metric	Imperial	US
25ml	1fl oz	
60ml	2fl oz	¼ cup
75ml	2½ fl oz	
100ml	3½fl oz	
120ml	4fl oz	½ cup
150ml	5fl oz	
175ml	6fl oz	
200ml	7fl oz	
250ml	8½ fl oz	1 cup
300ml	10½ fl oz	
360ml	12½ fl oz	
400ml	14fl oz	
450ml	15½ fl oz	
600ml	1 pint	
750ml	1¼ pint	3 cups
1 litre	1½ pints	4 cups

Other COOKNATION TITLES

If you enjoyed 'The Skinny 30 Minute Meals Recipe Book' we'd really appreciate your feedback. Reviews help others decide if this is the right book for them so a moment of your time would be appreciated.

Thank you.

You may also be interested in other '**Skinny**' titles in the CookNation series. You can find all the following great titles by searching under '**CookNation**'.

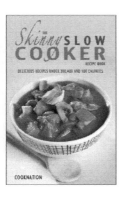

THE SKINNY SLOW COOKER RECIPE BOOK

Delicious Recipes Under 300, 400 And 500 Calories.

Paperback / eBook

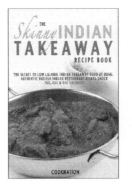

THE SKINNY INDIAN TAKEAWAY RECIPE BOOK

Authentic British Indian Restaurant Dishes Under 300, 400 And 500 Calories. The Secret To Low Calorie Indian Takeaway Food At Home.

Paperback / eBook

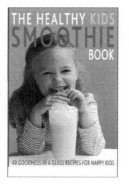

THE HEALTHY KIDS SMOOTHIE BOOK

40 Delicious Goodness In A Glass Recipes for Happy Kids.

eBook

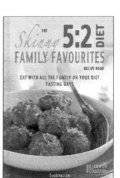

THE SKINNY 5:2 FAST DIET FAMILY FAVOURITES RECIPE BOOK

Eat With All The Family On Your Diet Fasting Days.

Paperback / eBook

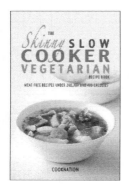

THE SKINNY SLOW COOKER VEGETARIAN RECIPE BOOK

40 Delicious Recipes Under 200, 300 And 400 Calories.

Paperback / eBook

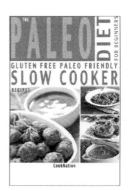

THE PALEO DIET FOR BEGINNERS SLOW COOKER RECIPE BOOK

Gluten Free, Everyday Essential Slow Cooker Paleo Recipes For Beginners.

eBook

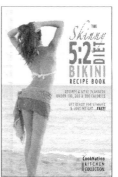
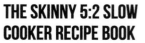
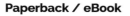

THE SKINNY 5:2 SLOW COOKER RECIPE BOOK

Skinny Slow Cooker Recipe And Menu Ideas Under 100, 200, 300 & 400 Calories For Your 5:2 Diet.

Paperback / eBook

THE SKINNY 5:2 BIKINI DIET RECIPE BOOK

Recipes & Meal Planners Under 100, 200 & 300 Calories. Get Ready For Summer & Lose Weight...FAST!

Paperback / eBook
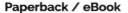

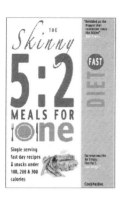

THE SKINNY 5:2 FAST DIET MEALS FOR ONE

Single Serving Fast Day Recipes & Snacks Under 100, 200 & 300 Calories.

Paperback / eBook

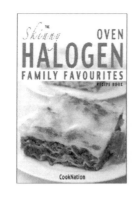

THE SKINNY HALOGEN OVEN FAMILY FAVOURITES RECIPE BOOK

Healthy, Low Calorie Family Meal-Time Halogen Oven Recipes Under 300, 400 and 500 Calories.

Paperback / eBook

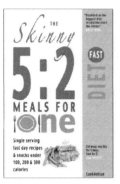

THE SKINNY 5:2 FAST DIET VEGETARIAN MEALS FOR ONE

Single Serving Fast Day Recipes & Snacks Under 100, 200 & 300 Calories.

Paperback / eBook

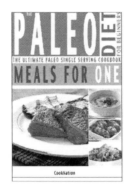

THE PALEO DIET FOR BEGINNERS MEALS FOR ONE

The Ultimate Paleo Single Serving Cookbook.

Paperback / eBook

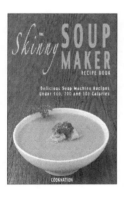

THE SKINNY SOUP MAKER RECIPE BOOK

Delicious Low Calorie, Healthy and Simple Soup Recipes Under 100, 200 and 300 Calories. Perfect For Any Diet and Weight Loss Plan.

Paperback / eBook

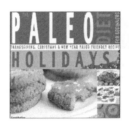

THE PALEO DIET FOR BEGINNERS HOLIDAYS

Thanksgiving, Christmas & New Year Paleo Friendly Recipes.
eBook

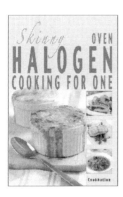

SKINNY HALOGEN OVEN COOKING FOR ONE

Single Serving, Healthy, Low Calorie Halogen Oven RecipesUnder 200, 300 and 400 Calories.

Paperback / eBook

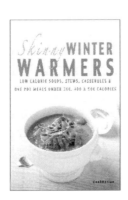

SKINNY WINTER WARMERS RECIPE BOOK

Soups, Stews, Casseroles & One Pot Meals Under 300, 400 & 500 Calories.

Paperback / eBook

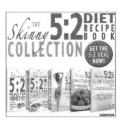

THE SKINNY 5:2 DIET RECIPE BOOK COLLECTION

All The 5:2 Fast Diet Recipes You'll Ever Need. All Under 100, 200, 300, 400 And 500 Calories.

eBook

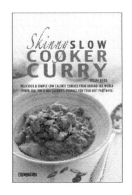

THE SKINNY SLOW COOKER CURRY RECIPE BOOK

Low Calorie Curries From Around The World.

Paperback / eBook

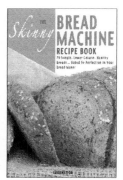

THE SKINNY BREAD MACHINE RECIPE BOOK

70 Simple, Lower Calorie, Healthy Breads...Baked To Perfection In Your Bread Maker.

Paperback / eBook

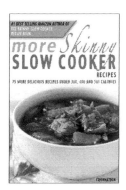

MORE SKINNY SLOW COOKER RECIPES

75 More Delicious Recipes Under 300, 400 & 500 Calories.

Paperback / eBook

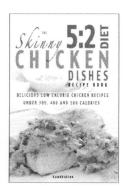

THE SKINNY 5:2 DIET CHICKEN DISHES RECIPE BOOK

Delicious Low Calorie Chicken Dishes Under 300, 400 & 500 Calories.

Paperback / eBook

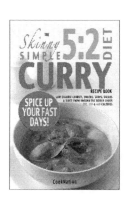

THE SKINNY 5:2 CURRY RECIPE BOOK

Spice Up Your Fast Days With Simple Low Calorie Curries, Snacks, Soups, Salads & Sides Under 200, 300 & 400 Calories.

Paperback / eBook

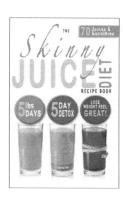

THE SKINNY JUICE DIET RECIPE BOOK

5lbs, 5 Days. The Ultimate Kick- Start Diet and Detox Plan to Lose Weight & Feel Great!

Paperback / eBook

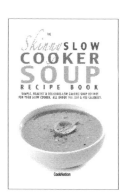

THE SKINNY SLOW COOKER SOUP RECIPE BOOK

Simple, Healthy & Delicious Low Calorie Soup Recipes For Your Slow Cooker. All Under 100, 200 & 300 Calories.

Paperback / eBook

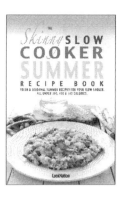

THE SKINNY SLOW COOKER SUMMER RECIPE BOOK

Fresh & Seasonal Summer Recipes For Your Slow Cooker. All Under 300, 400 And 500 Calories.

Paperback / eBook

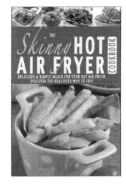

THE SKINNY HOT AIR FRYER COOKBOOK

Delicious & Simple Meals For Your Hot Air Fryer: Discover The Healthier Way To Fry.

Paperback / eBook

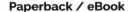
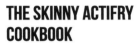

THE SKINNY ACTIFRY COOKBOOK

Guilt-free and Delicious ActiFry Recipe Ideas: Discover The Healthier Way to Fry!

Paperback / eBook

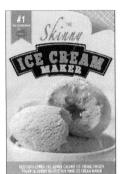

THE SKINNY ICE CREAM MAKER

Delicious Lower Fat, Lower Calorie Ice Cream, Frozen Yogurt & Sorbet Recipes For Your Ice Cream Maker.

Paperback / eBook

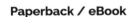

THE SKINNY 15 MINUTE MEALS RECIPE BOOK

Delicious, Nutritious & Super-Fast Meals in 15 Minutes Or Less. All Under 300, 400 & 500 Calories.

Paperback / eBook

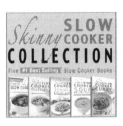

THE SKINNY SLOW COOKER COLLECTION

5 Fantastic Books of Delicious, Diet-friendly Skinny Slow Cooker Recipes: ALL Under 200, 300, 400 & 500 Calories!
eBook

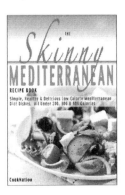

THE SKINNY MEDITERRANEAN RECIPE BOOK

Simple, Healthy & Delicious Low Calorie Mediterranean Diet Dishes. All Under 200, 300 & 400 Calories.

Paperback / eBook

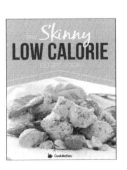

THE SKINNY LOW CALORIE RECIPE BOOK

Great Tasting, Simple & Healthy Meals Under 300, 400 & 500 Calories. Perfect For Any Calorie Controlled Diet.

Paperback / eBook

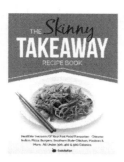

THE SKINNY TAKEAWAY RECIPE BOOK

Healthier Versions Of Your Fast Food Favourites: All Under 300, 400 & 500 Calories.

Paperback / eBook

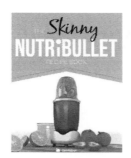

THE SKINNY NUTRIBULLET RECIPE BOOK

80+ Delicious & Nutritious Healthy Smoothie Recipes. Burn Fat, Lose Weight and Feel Great!

Paperback / eBook

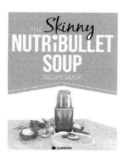

THE SKINNY NUTRIBULLET SOUP RECIPE BOOK

Delicious, Quick & Easy, Single Serving Soups & Pasta Sauces For Your Nutribullet. All Under 100, 200, 300 & 400 Calories!

Paperback / eBook

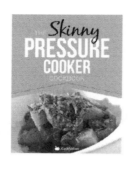

THE SKINNY PRESSURE COOKER COOKBOOK

USA ONLY

Low Calorie, Healthy & Delicious Meals, Sides & Desserts. All Under 300, 400 & 500 Calories.

Paperback / eBook

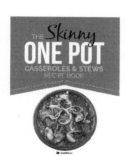

THE SKINNY ONE-POT RECIPE BOOK

Simple & Delicious, One-Pot Meals. All Under 300, 400 & 500 Calories

Paperback / eBook

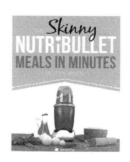

THE SKINNY NUTRIBULLET MEALS IN MINUTES RECIPE BOOK

Quick & Easy, Single Serving Suppers, Snacks, Sauces, Salad Dressings & More Using Your Nutribullet. All Under 300, 400 & 500 Calories

Paperback / eBook

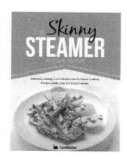

THE SKINNY STEAMER RECIPE BOOK

Healthy, Low Calorie, Low Fat Steam Cooking Recipes Under 300, 400 & 500 Calories.

Paperback / eBook

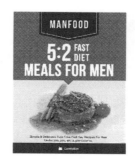

MANFOOD: 5:2 FAST DIET MEALS FOR MEN

Simple & Delicious, Fuss Free, Fast Day Recipes For Men Under 200, 300, 400 & 500 Calories.

Paperback / eBook

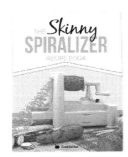

THE SKINNY SPIRALIZER RECIPE BOOK

Delicious Spiralizer Inspired Low Calorie Recipes For One. All Under 200, 300, 400 & 500 Calories

Paperback / eBook

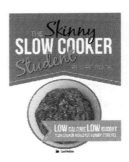

THE SKINNY SLOW COOKER STUDENT RECIPE BOOK

Delicious, Simple, Low Calorie, Low Budget, Slow Cooker Meals For Hungry Students. All Under 300, 400 & 500 Calories

Paperback / eBook

12036615R00055

Printed in Great Britain
by Amazon.co.uk, Ltd.,
Marston Gate.